GIVE IT ONE MORE TRY

CLARENCE KD MCNAIR

ISBN-13: 978-1-7341797-2-9

This book was printed in the United States of America

To order additional copies of this book contact:
LaBoo Publishing Enterprise, LLC
staff@laboopublishing.com
www.laboopublishing.com

To book the author contact:
info@mcnairbooks.com

Table of Contents

Dedication

This book is dedicated to all of the overcomers in the world who were one step away from giving up. I hope this book transforms your mind from any negative thought that can alter your life. To my two children, Khori and Amaria, I hope you learn from me so you can take a different route towards greatness. Special dedication to my wife Tracy McNair: you have been encouraging me to focus on my gifts and share my story with the world. I appreciate you more than you will ever know.

Acknowledgments

THANK YOU FOR HELPING ME COMMIT TO MY PURPOSE

I want to thank God for giving me the talent, ability and vision to create great work. To my family and supporters, thank you for the good and bad times that shaped who I am today. Without those experiences of negativity and dysfunction, I wouldn't have the wisdom I need to help people today. I especially thank my mom for opening the door to a whole new world in my younger days and making the sacrifices that you made that helped me get to where I am today. To my stepfather, thanks for riding this journey with us even though the road was really bumpy from time to time. I also want to thank my father; you may not have been in my life, but from a distance you taught me the ability to get through anything. Because of you, I've learned a valuable lesson of persistence. I want to thank my younger brother Antoine and older sister Francine for being great. I know you both have endured many ups and downs, yet you never gave up and continuously give life one more try no matter what life may bring.

I want to thank Ciara Suesberry, also known as Berry Dynamic, for your commitment. To my respiratory therapist, Kecia, thank you for your kind support and encouragement. Janie Cauthorne, thank you for always reminding me to put myself first. Thank you Pinky Cole, for encouraging me to tell my story. Thank you Karlie Redd, for always listening to my one million ideas even if we only nailed one. I really appreciate your ear and your belief in me.

Special thanks to the Gayle family for your support, and to my cousin Nathaniel Mercer for always seeing the light at the end of the tunnel, even when no one believed there was a tunnel. To my prayer warrior Jerome Lattisaw, thank you for opening your house up to me when I had nowhere to go, and my soldier Ferman Barnes, thank you for always believing in me from day one. Thank you Amber Ravenel for believing in my talents; even when things would fall through, you still believed in me. Thank you Shay Star, for never turning your back on me, no matter what. Thank you Jay Reezy for your patience. Thank you Dr. George and Benjamin for helping me to gain my life back. Thank you Jesse McDade, for sharing your talent and grooming me from the start. I could go on and on, but to every person who ever invested in my life, spoke life into my life, prayed for me and loved me, thank you.

Introduction

If you picked up this book, hopefully you're thinking about giving it one more try. I know I did, and that's why I wrote this book: to help someone, and I hope that someone is you. After reading this book you will gain a newfound respect for the things that did not work out in your life. I hope that through my story and what I've learned, you will see your failures, your let downs, and disappointments as tools to better yourself, to get back up, and to "give it one more try," but this time seeing those failures and heartaches as stepping stones, a training experience for what God has for you next. Remember, life is all about second chances, so do not let your second chance go out the door without fighting for it. Now grab some tea or coffee and walk with me as I take you on a journey with me to happy, and at the end, I hope you will find a reason to smile again.

CHAPTER ONE

Winning to Lose

In order for you to understand my story, I have to share how the obstacles in my life were used for good. Absolutely nothing was given to me, I had to fight for my life in order to have the life I have today. I am a survivor of anxiety who suffered greatly from the war within me. Not knowing how to set myself free, I exhausted my ability to fight and had no idea how to unlock my destiny. With a million things to do and people depending on me, my life revolved around others' happiness. I held the keys of prosperity, yet seemed to have misplaced mine. On the outside, I was KD: The world's musical artist and recording manager. On the inside, Clarence was losing it. Somewhere in between, I was battling with myself.

I couldn't remember the last time – or even the first time – I asked for help. It was the moment when fear and pride battled within me, and I accepted the fact that winners lose too. When it happened, it was a hard loss I couldn't fathom. My truth of suppressed hurtful memories began to reveal themselves. The smile I wore disguised the different world I lived within. Eventually, my mental health mysteriously began to fail and I knew I couldn't hide it anymore. Everything was hitting me at once, and I was wrestling to get out of a sunken place.

Music has always been my first love. Growing up in East Baltimore, Maryland, I witnessed everybody hurting to survive. Born with a collapsed kidney, I was introduced to pain very early in life. Stereotypes were real. Most kids grew up without their fathers; mine was taken away by the system. Twenty-five years of my life was spent learning how to understand something that took me 30 years to accomplish. The jail visits at nine years old to see my father aroused much confusion. Struggling to understand why my pops stayed away from home introduced psychological trauma into my life and made my racing mind dangerous. Mom was my biggest supporter in life, but was sometimes not the easiest person to talk to or interact with. At times she was jittery, moving fast and searching for balance, which in turn made me nervous. Amongst us all, I felt like my mom had the hardest time dealing with my father going to prison; she'd experienced her two brothers going to jail and my father was another man taken away from her, leaving her a single-mother to raise two kids. Mom worked at Johns Hopkins Hospital scrubbing floors and cleaning toilets to keep food in our stomachs and the lights on. My mother, oldest sister and I were having some tough times until my mom remarried to my stepfather, which brought us better support.

We were literally just getting by while tribulation successfully ran its course through my family. A few years later, my granny stopped working because her health began to fail her. To assist my mom with my siblings and I, we often spent nights with our granny who lived in the projects. As much as I loved my granny, I dreaded the car rides to her house, because of our adopted cousin who lived there. Once getting past the indecent exposure and unpleasant experiences, my memories at Granny's house were unforgettable. Back then, all of the children had to sleep in one room. It was very awkward waking up in the middle of the night hearing my cousin on the phone with his girlfriend, fondling himself in the same bed we all slept in. To top that off, he was the same cousin who teased me growing up. Calling me a fagot, he would pull on me by my underwear and try to kiss me on my face. I just remember being afraid of him, never knowing what to expect. I told my granny about him picking on me and being unsure around him.

Being surrounded by people with emotional disorders stirred up unnecessary chaos I didn't ask for. My family was truly going through the storm and only God could save us. First, there was my uncle whose life seemed to go downhill after he stepped on a rusty nail. He began to experience health issues, eating uncontrollably, vomiting everywhere and having nervous breakdowns without his medication. For the longest time, I thought he was just crazy until I learned he hadn't always been that way. The stiff hand of cards he was dealt in life caused his mind to spin out of control.

My other uncle went through a phase of giving up for whatever reason I couldn't understand. He was usually the levelheaded uncle I could talk to about regular teenage experiences. Although his comments were rarely given in conversations, it was cool to have somebody who was interested in hearing about my day. Things changed when he decided he was done listening to people. One day, he rushed into the house upset and straight into the bathroom. Noticing him in my peripheral, his pacing and random mid-day bath made me rather uneasy. The gloomy look on his face was incomprehensible as he slowly shut and locked the door. Immediately, my spirit didn't feel right: his frequency felt too low. My other uncle, his brother, just so happened to walk by the door where he heard the water overflowing onto the floor and soaking the hallway carpet. Before I knew it, I could hear family members screaming, kicking, bombarding and yelling his name to open the door. Preparing for the conditions on the other side, the suspense of whether his life could be saved or if he would be pronounced dead awaited us all. Lifting his body from the tub, the resuscitation process began immediately and was the most intense three minutes of my life. Hearing the gasp of his revived body gave us all hope, and that was the day I learned about suicide. It taught me how one's environment can make or break them. This determines the mental stability of a person and demonstrates their ability to handle a situation. It was amazing to see what the power of fighting for what's rightfully yours can accomplish. My uncle was drowning, but the people around him refused to let him die. No matter how jacked up our living terms were, nobody was allowed to leave this earth a coward. Eventually, the same uncle was arrested and sentenced to over 10 years in jail for robbery. After he was released, he was rebirthed and given another try at life, more time to figure it out, and an extra chance to make something out of himself.

More fear was placed into my heart the first time I felt a gun pressed against my back. From this time on, stress got the best of me and walks to school never felt safe again. It was like I was getting attacked from all angles and the closest people in my life couldn't protect me because they were agonized with their own drama. From childhood into my adult life, I experienced many challenges. My aunt had bad nerves and worried about everything. My oldest sister was going to jail every other weekend. By this time, my father was getting out of jail for the first time and was living with my sister. Then I was moving in with them after my divorce. Once we all were situated, my sister was going back to jail and was up for a 30-year hearing. Together, dysfunction was our normal way of living.

Thinking back on the different moments in life, I had to find coping mechanisms to escape from the tragedies I endured. Through it all, my vivid imagination helped me follow my dreams and ignite my passions. Speaking things into existence was instilled into me at a young age. Because music was my gift, talent shows were my version of concerts, giving me the freedom to pour my heart onto the stage. Although I was disturbed by everything happening to and around me, I knew I needed to operate in the mindset of how I wanted to live and not adapt to the way I was living. Reminiscing on my childhood, my teacher would tell my mom how I would daydream in class about caviar on the rocks, Hollywood, and all things that seemed far-fetched at the time. I still remember the Michael Jackson outfit my mother handmade with safety pins all over the jacket, old black penny loafers, high water black slacks, with the infamous sequined white glove. I walked out onto the stage confident, ready to reveal my alter-ego Bootsie. When the beat dropped, I knew then I was born to be a star. I exhaled every fearful bone in my body and gave my all. I closed the show with the epic spin and left every emotion on the stage. When my name was called as the first-place winner, I knew I needed to feel that way forever; it was the most profound moment in my life.

From that day on, my mom made sure I traveled to New York frequently to increase my exposure. Maxing out her credit cards, she motivated me to make sure my music was something people needed to hear. She was using her resources to make ends meet and I appreciated every investment she put into me. Even though it stressed her out, the support meant the world to me. My first cassette tape self-entitled "Bootsie" dropped in 1994. I was 16 years old dropping music reflecting my thoughts with pop and R&B vibes. My first song was "It Feels Like Magic in The Air." After graduating from Patterson High School in 1996, my gift for music was recognized by Brian Dickens, who my mom and I met at the "For Sisters Only Expo." He was known for working with K-CI & JOJO, Yolanda Adams and a stream of other gospel artists. He gave me a chance to prove myself worthy.

Through Brian Dickens, I was introduced to Stacy Lattisaw's brother Jerome, also known as Goldie, a huge R&B musician in the '80s, and was given his number on a sheet of paper. I'd just enrolled into Essex Community College in Baltimore. After meeting Jerome Lattisaw, I dropped out of college after a week to pursue my music career full time. Shortly after, I ended up losing Goldie's number for three months. Facebook and Instagram didn't exist back then, so if you lost somebody's number, that was it. Feeling like a huge opportunity had slipped right through my fingers, my spirits were crushed. Things didn't go the way I had expected them to, and I constantly hoped God would make a way. They say if you want to find something, stop looking for it. When I finally did, my mom ended up finding Goldie's number on a sheet of paper in the couch while cleaning the house. When I say prayers are real, that's the truth because there was no way something like that should have happened. However, good things come to those who wait. The call to Goldie was a life-changing experience as he couldn't wait to hear the music. We sent the demo, signed a major recording contract with Haqq Islam, CEO of University Records/Interscope Records, and the rest was history. Majusty, later named Prophet Jones, our first demo was placed in the soundtrack for Jamie Foxx's movie *Bait*. We were now amongst the roster of notable artists such as Missy Elliot, Mya, Nelly, Donell Jones, and Fat Joe. After a few years of being signed on the Interscope label, Haqq Islam and Steve Stoute, who at the time was President of Black Music, had a major falling out, which ended our deal with Interscope.

Can you imagine being 19 years old, snatched from the inner cities of Baltimore, and in the blink of an eye going from eating rations to three-course meals every day? "I made it out" was my thought. After the first deal, with the assistance of Haqq Islam and Russell Simmons, founder of Def Jam Records, Prophet Jones became a part of history. We signed our contract with the legendary Motown Records, a company successful for launching the biggest artists ever known, such as Michael Jackson, The Jackson Five, Marvin Gaye and The Temptations. I was at the peak of my career! Prophet Jones was opening shows for Mya, Sisqo, Ruff Ryders, Jagged Edge, Brian McKnight, Eve and many more. We also starred on Soul Train with Shemar Moore, Master P, and Christina Milian. The best experience I remember was headlining and appearing on MTV2 and BET's 106th & Park with hosts AJ and Free. That was a big moment for my family to see me on National TV for the first time. Not to mention, the press was going crazy! One of the coolest memories with my group members was standing on stage with other artists like Whitney Houston, Sean "P. Diddy" Combs, and religious leader Louis Farrakhan at the Million Family March in the year 2000 in Washington D.C. We obtained press placements in *Vibe*, *Billboard*, *Sister 2 Sister* and *Seventeen* magazines. Prophet Jones appeared on the BET game show *On the Beat* in 2001 along with DJ LaLa Anthony, currently the wife of NBA Star and Baltimore native Carmelo Anthony. Then, we were later featured in *Jet Magazine* on the 2002 Top 10 Albums of the Year list along with Michael Jackson. Yes, Michael Jackson! In 2004, we traveled to Tokyo to perform for the United States Military Troops.

We were the movers and shakers of the early 2000s and God had answered my prayers. For the first time, I felt like I could be the man of the house and was happy to provide for my family whenever they needed something. I had beat the system and began to give my family everything they ever dreamed of. It was literally Christmas all up and through Baltimore, and I never thought twice about the high I was on: Successful. As a recording artist, I worked with video director Gil Green, who serviced platinum artists such as Lil Wayne, Rick Ross, Akon and the infamous video director Jessy Terrero. Things really hit the climax once the opportunity appeared to work with Jazze Pha (producer for Ciara), McKelly Jamison (producer for Faith Evans and Carl Thomas), Grammy Award Winning Songwriter Gordon Chambers, Philadelphia's legendary songwriters Gamble and Huff, as well as the production team of Tricky Stewart from Red Zone Entertainment, who produced artists such as Rihanna and Beyonce.

Never allow yourself to get so successful that you forget the value of life itself. Sometimes, God has a way of bringing you back to the natural state of a humbling mindset. As I was on the all-time high of my life, my failure awaited to plan its sneak attack of depression. Out of the blue, Prophet Jones' deal went bad and my career hit rock bottom in 2002. I lost an advance of 125K towards my second album, which Motown Records wanted to produce. Motown was so upset with the situation that they shipped my previous records to the house. In addition, my accolades were stripped of value and everything I worked hard for became irrelevant. The life was literally sucked away from me; music was all I ever knew. I went from having the worldwide recognition as Motown Records' hit male R&B singer with three record deals to nothing for a long period of time. The worst part about being dropped from the label was not knowing. I was still making investments and pouring my all into an album nobody was going to hear. I was booking shows for an audience that wouldn't see me perform. I was the star of the ultimate joke. Coming home with nothing was the most terrifying moment of my life, right next to becoming homeless.

Once my faith was challenged, it was up to me to climb over the tallest mountain in my life. The person I thought I was no longer existed, and I slipped into a dark place. We went from living in condos in Manhattan, five-star restaurant dining, purchasing the desires of our hearts to being right back at square one. I was the man who failed his family and it tore me up on the inside. I allowed the enemy to destroy my mind, which forced me to pray harder because now my life truly depended on it. It was at that moment that I had to remember who I was and how far I'd come after losing it all.

Not admitting to needing help is the first sign of self-neglect. Most of us lock away our truth and forget we are the same ones who hold the key. Keeping everything bottled in was the harshest thing I could've done to my body. Memories resurfaced, present circumstances overwhelmed me, and not knowing the outcome of my future destroyed my everything. Stress is the biggest silent killer. Beware of withholding traumatic experiences, feelings and thoughts inside because it has a tendency to reveal itself in the most unexpected ways. For me, I began losing my appetite, losing sleep, isolating myself from social environments, devaluing my self-worth and confidence, and developed major body aches. Little did I know, my body was sending signs that something wasn't right. When we fail to share and open up about the trials of life, we become our own enemy when we battle against our own emotions. The worst thing a person can do is keep their minds busy with never-ending to-do lists. Because this allows us to hide who we are, we internally are stagnating our mental ability to address the real issues kept within. Ultimately, don't forget to love yourself and be open about your struggles. This will decrease your stress levels, create opportunities for you to heal, and truly take control of your identity and purpose in life.

CHAPTER TWO

Fearing to Lose

Some of us give too much power to fear, especially when we're comfortable at rock bottom. Challenges arrive and one day you're starting from square one. Having no clue what waited for my tomorrows, it drove me insane. Everything became an asset to determine how much further I would fall into the pit or how much closer I was to coming out of it. To be at the peak of my career then suddenly homeless, my mind immediately reverted back to my childhood. I began to remember the long nights of emotional stress and channel the success of my failure. Applying for disability because of my anxiety was the moment I gave fear too much power. I realized fear tried to step in and have its way with me, and I almost let it get away with my happiness.

With very few resources, I was a child again; carless, broke, without a pot to piss in and a window to throw it out of. I was back in the midst of dysfunction and had to stare at it every day. This time, it was in my control. There were times I felt like my heart was going to bust out of my chest in the middle of the highway.

Driving to no destination with a racing mind reminded me of my life; living without a destination. That alone made my mental stability weaker. Before I knew it, I was suffering from insomnia, losing unhealthy amounts of weight, and rushing to the emergency room five times a month. My EKG tests, full body X-rays, and blood work all came back healthy. The conclusion was that my mind was at war! My symptoms included panic attacks, anxiety disorder, and heart palpitations. It took a while to come to terms with the fact that I was mentally ill and suffering from severe anxiety and depression.

Beginning to understand the psychology behind anxiety will help people know how to properly react to situations. A healthy community will represent positive influencers and comfortable living, In the typical African American household, these types of problems are hardly ever acknowledged to exist. In actuality, however, this disorder is very common in our communities due to the oppression and poverty we are constantly exposed to. Instead of our environments being free of violence, we tend to adjust to our circumstance or surroundings, instead of accurately dealing with the issues. I couldn't remember the last time somebody asked me if I was okay or offered to genuinely pray for me. My mind was literally exploding and only I could feel the ooze dripping from my ear. Hearing the negativity, seeing the disappointments, feeling my heart take it all in, and coming to terms with not being okay took its toll on me. Anxiety has a way of making a person self-medicate. Developing an addictive appetite, I understood the risks in why some people smoke a pack of cigarettes a day or depend of retail therapy to make them feel better. This was the power of drugs, sex, crime, alcohol and food. However, I self-medicated through finding love. This is something that people should refrain from because you'll find yourself further compromising your happiness to not be alone. Remember, you are typically not in your right mind, so you depend on that person to heal your sorrows. This is not good for a healthy relationship, and you build your forever on broken ground.

On top of that, I was struggling financially. We've been taught to believe the love of money is the root of all evil. I believe the lack of money is. It's the reason why we break our backs and the bank to reach our goals, or for some, the reason why we hurt people. Thinking back, my mom went bankrupt helping me secure my music career. She was $75,000 in the hole before I signed a one-million-dollar record deal. Realizing what had been sacrificed, giving up wasn't an option. As an adult, the IRS was constantly on my back and claimed I owed them $32,000. Can you imagine how stressful this is? Knowing that every check you earn doesn't belong to you. What's even crazier is when people won't use their saved money to invest and create better situations for themselves. Life has tricked us into becoming a slave to the illusion of money, instead of making our dollars a slave to our passions. I personally believe another reason why we suffer from mental health is because we hold on to our currency rather than investing it into something that's going to advance. Realistically, if all you have is money, then you are poor. But if you have land, you are richer than any person you contact.

When you are mentally unstable, nothing will make sense and you have to accept the fact of needing help. Speaking to a psychiatrist was hard, but worth it. At the time, I was prescribed medication to cope with my anxiety. Psychologically, I was overcoming anxiety. Opening up about the spiteful moments in my life, I reconnected with God on a spiritual level and truly began my process of healing. I know seeking counseling is not considered the ideal solution within the community I was raised in, but I needed to get the understanding of why I went through certain things. I needed to transform my way of coping with pain. Although not everyone may agree with this method, it gave me the medical help I unconsciously yearned for. The solution was to collectively change the way I lived my life. This included balance. First, we must recognize our body as a temple and treat it as such. Everything we digest, whether it's food, knowledge, or energy, has an effect on our bodies. Exercising played a huge role in how I strengthened my mind on a regular basis. Eating right was equally as important because psychologically, we are what we eat. Our minds are controlled through the food we take in. Increasing my intake of fruits and vegetables, while abstaining from sodium and alcohol, allowed my body to improve. God was making a change in my life, motivating me to be a better and healthier man. All I had to do was truly allow him into my life.

This is when you get to the core of what's causing the problem. Vulnerability was the key. You have to make a decision that you want to live, which requires you to speak life into your life. Beware of your surroundings, your circle of influence, the thoughts you absorb, and the door you choose to walk through. Realizing you are the key and only you can unlock your destiny to freedom. The truth is the padlock on the door. However, we sometimes allow distractions to keep us from unlocking the truth. We overwhelm ourselves with what others will think and how they will judge us. Thus, we must always find the willpower to pick ourselves up, turn the padlock to our life, and open the door to prosperity. Don't give in to depression and anxiety, fight for your existence and take everything that comes along with being transparent.

Truth be told, only God can give you peace. Sometimes, He gives us trials and tribulations to handle in life to challenge our faith in him. Everything from there becomes a test. Win or lose, you have to never play yourself. Today, I am able to handle failures differently as a wise man versus when I was younger. I view the obstacles in life as a way of iron sharpening iron. Having money, a particular image, and materialistic things don't make you successful; having joy, happiness, value, a clearer vision of life and your dignity does. Everything else is a bonus. Often times, people get caught up in the lifestyle of success, but don't know how to maintain their sanity through it all. I want to help other people learn how to manage both.

It's not often people fail, succeed, fail again, then bounce back successfully ten times over. After Prophet Jones, I started turning my gift into profit by consulting people needing brand management and creative direction. To this day, I'm glad it worked out in my favor because at that time I knew a regular nine-to-five wasn't going to cut it for me. I was loyal to R&B music and needed to be free to operate in a creative space. To flourish in my expertise, I took every skill I learned as an artist and became the teacher. Hard work earned me the title of a recording manager, an entertainment consultant for several projects, an adviser for many songwriters, and a concert promoter. What can I say? I redeemed myself and began to hold the key to everyone's destiny. All I had to do was turn the lock.

CHAPTER THREE

Coping with Isolation

When my father was released from prison, he was homeless for a few months. Every day, I had to gather myself mentally to bring him food under the bridge. In order to truly know if you've overcome a situation, sometimes you have to stare into its eyes. It was the toughest moment because it reminded me of how I felt as a child wishing my father could come home. It reminded me of how it tore me up seeing my father get high. It reminded me that our family's provider wasn't stable and was near giving up. This moment humbled me, allowing me to properly reflect on the time when I myself was partially homeless after Prophet Jones and had to move back home with my mom. Yet, it almost destroyed me as a man to see my father in this condition. This was God's reminder to never quit and be grateful of your transformation.

Your circle of influence has a major effect on the mind, more than you think. Witnessing my oldest sister with shackles around her hands and ankles reminded me of slavery and hurt me to the core when we visited her. Watching my mom leave her job to take care of my little sister, and hearing her complain and fuss all the time because we had no money, increased my stress levels. Going with my youngest sister to the doctor to get CT scans and watching her break down the day I dropped her off at college because of her condition enhanced my headaches and made me cry many times. My stepfather married my mother to mend her broken heart, until he became exhausted trying to love her. I believe my mom was dealing with so much internally and didn't get the help she needed before committing to him. It was painful to watch him stop fighting for her. After I had my son, I remembered what it felt like to not have my father; not having a strong relationship with him mentally drained me. The frequent disagreements with my son's mother and being threatened with jail time because of arrears in child support disturbed my heart, when all I wanted to do in my heart was co-parent. Collectively, it's hard to see your family constantly on the battlefield. The great part about our situation was that our family had nine lives. We could never be broken. This is when the will to never give up becomes very crucial. Taking it all in, I realized pushing through was all that mattered.

Technically, there's no way in the world I should be able to tell you my story right now. When your trials don't kill you, they make you stronger and able to share your testimony with the world. This has pushed me to give life one more try, over and over again. For as long as I could remember, I carried my family's sorrows on my back and it all affected me negatively. The only thing I regret is my lack of urgency in taking my mental health seriously. My mental capacity for stress began to overflow; I couldn't stop no matter what. In life, you will get beat, hit with many blows, spit on, jabbed, walked on, but you can't give up. This is why the movie *Rocky* was a classic. He symbolized victory against adversity.

When you are mentally unstable, every opportunity will seem like a great opportunity until you distinguish between the people wanting to help you versus those who want to keep you held down. However, you must not allow these people to keep you from walking in your purpose. Remember, God gives his toughest missions to his true soldiers, so understand why you must go through trials. For me, I needed to be the Rocky in my family, so God could use me as a vessel. By doing so, I was able to accept Him being the one in control, and allow myself to merely control how I see and handle adversity.

The best moment of my life was when I hit rock bottom. It was the time when I didn't have any friends, so I befriended myself. This time of isolation birthed self-discovery using my secret weapon: prayer. Now when I talk about prayer, it's not the typical "just go pray about it" response I'm giving you. We must first learn how to pray correctly. Prayer is what you tell yourself, how you speak to God, what you expect out of life and how it empowers you to help others. This is the moment to truly speak positivity into existence and not focus so much on the negativity of the present. You have to understand that most things don't last forever, not even the hardships of our daily life. Just as people gossip or curse, people can take that same energy and transform it into a powerful prayer. This was the only thing that kept me able to function appropriately and maintain a healthy mindset after battling with my own demons.

Understand, this will take time. Once, I was under so much anxiety from engulfing everyone's problems including mine. I was young, married, and searching for answers through religion. My woman at the time was practicing a different religion from how I was raised, which made me unconsciously separate myself from my family. I was going to the Kingdom Hall and following their ways of belief. Even though I battled against the teachings stored within, I learned more about God from a different perspective. I glorified their unity, until I began to see that everybody has problems regardless of their background. Jumping from one extreme to the next, I was digging myself into a deeper hole. I was truly lost and just wanted to have a place to call home. The moral of my story is to never seek solutions in other human beings; you'll get disappointed every time because no one is perfect. However, I learned so many helpful things about life going to the Kingdom Hall.

CHAPTER FOUR

Coping with Fear

Sometimes you need bricks on your back to build your back stronger, forcing you to tap into your supernatural human abilities. Just as our muscles can lose mass and become weak when unused, we must tolerate pressure to know how to react to life's hardships. This activates our survivor mode to help us grow as individuals. The truth is, we have so many statistics to overtake, so many expectations to exceed. By acknowledging the stones in life known as problems, we must leverage every boulder as steps towards victory. Without doing so, we will only lead ourselves towards mental illness and forever struggle to maintain healthy lifestyles.

None of our stories will be the same. However, our circumstances will cause us to undergo the symptoms of anxiety at some point in life. Because seeking counseling is viewed as being mentally incompetent, we internally hurt ourselves even more when we suppress these feelings. Be determined to not become your own enemy. Listening to motivational videos was how I trained my mind to combat the negative thoughts of self-defeat. I spent hours at Barnes and Nobles Bookstore reading various anxiety books, comprehending how our characteristics play a role in how we approach life. I realized fear was used for controlling purposes and how it ignited my anxiety attacks. When I was not in control of my reactions, I gave power to every situation that bothered me. I devoted years searching for that big moment that would change my life and put me back on top of the world. I wanted to feel like I did when I was on stage sharing my feelings. To complement my journey, I began studying food by eliminating little things out of my diet like dairy, sugar, chocolate, potato chips, and started cooking my food in olive oil. This helped me understand the power of mentally digesting what I physically ingested, and the significance of water and proper rest.

My favorite part of my journey was learning about how visualization relaxation can imminently heal the mind. Visualization relaxation encouraged me to walk daily and become one with nature. In the environment of what's considered the "ghetto," some of the community members tend to be stressed or surrounded by negativity; whereas people who live in nice communities surrounding lakes have a better chance of being peaceful, happy, and stable. I realized that environmental visuals played a huge role in my childhood and how I mentally felt about myself. Visuals are a key component in psychology. This explains why vacation resorts are so profitable, or even homes that are more expensive by the water, because you are literally paying for the visuals; peace to relax the mind and body. It works the same with the kind of car we drive; it reflects ourselves and state of living. Ultimately, anything that plays a role in causing anxiety and unhealthy chemical reactions must be eradicated before it leads to an influence, to self-destruction.

CHAPTER FIVE

Leave Life Alone, Let It Be

Most of us turn away from peace because we turn away from what's supernatural. As time goes by, you tend to realize when you must let things be. Once I lost everything at the age of 25, I stopped being true to myself. I stopped writing music, socially interacting with people, and eventually stopped using my gifts. I allowed depression to cave down on me. I stopped being creative and growing into the person God ordained for me to be. It took years for me to get back to myself and a total of 15 years to realize the principles I was going to live by for the rest of my life.

The following are these principles.

1. **Put Yourself First**: Whether it's taking better care of yourself, eating properly, exercising, following your hobbies, pursuing your career or passion, do it first. Often times, people get caught up in their situations and forget they have the power to change their circumstances for better or worse. Before you know it, you've created

this long list of things to-do with not a single thing relevant to your future. No matter what life throws at you, don't allow people to yank you up and down like a yo-yo. You were born with freedom and should always choose to control the flow of your life. You walk into a restaurant to wait in the long line and see a seat at the bar that you could sit at, rather than asking the group if the seat is taken, you hesitate and waste time making assumptions. You later see someone walk up to the same seat you were looking at and politely sit down after asking if she could sit there. Besides thinking that they were maybe saving the seat for a friend, you counted yourself out of an opportunity because you didn't put yourself first. Remember, the things you tell yourself determine the next moves toward your destiny.

2. **Build a community around your life**: The only way to hold yourself accountable in certain aspects of life is by affiliating with the right people. This is based on your circle of influence. There will be people in your life who will come to distract and discourage you from accomplishing your goals. These will be the people who will x themselves out of your life. People who don't understand your vision will laugh at you and try to play the "I told you so" role to make you believe they were right when you fail the tenth time. Comments like "You still trying to do that?" and "If it hasn't happened by now, then you might as well quit" constantly drilled into my mind. It

was up to me to understand and realize that in the midst of walking in your purpose, there will be times when all you hear is negativity. However, stay focused and beware not to consume pessimistic views nor become a believer of other people's fear and lack of faith. Just accept the fact that you're going to go through hell while on this journey to success. Most of all, it's going to be frustrating, and at times it'll make you feel misplaced on the inside. After losing my record deal, I went through a type of pain that felt worse than somebody dying. Even with losing a few family members in one year before, nothing hurt worse than losing a life-changing opportunity, because I felt like I let everybody down, including the members who passed away. Ultimately, it put me in an incompetent mind-frame that I wouldn't wish on anybody. Some people will get negative about your success and show their true colors. When people don't show you, they're happy for you, that's when your association with them becomes a problem. Don't find yourself having to flex on people to remind them of your credentials.

3. **Have a realistic perspective on life**: After hitting rock bottom, I learned how to mentally pull myself together by seeing my situation for its truth. I had to fight to gain my confidence, energy, happiness and determination back. Once this was accomplished, it helped me find reasons to be grateful and understand that success has nothing to do with money. Success is about overcoming

the challenges and roadblocks in life. People who have been in jail, have no job or can't seem to get anywhere are people who are usually in a negative space. This is also common in relationships. A man leaves his girlfriend of nine years for another woman, which causes her to jump into another relationship she's not ready for. After leaving all of that rut and anxiety, she didn't take time to heal and recover from the heartache. Instead, she jumped into another relationship and attracted the same type of man. Truth is, it takes time to look at a situation from a holistic aspect. Our environments play a huge role in how we perceive things in life. All in all, you have to be brand new in order to attract new energy. You have to get into a position where you simply want to give it one more try. This is possible by getting your mind right, which may require you to read the right books and take time to invest in yourself. Understand that you are a reflection of what you digest. Regardless of your environment, never settle for the way things may seem now; find a way to get into a positive mindset. This takes effort. You might have to drive to the library, or catch a bus to a quiet coffee shop or even go on a walk to another city if you feel it's worth it. If you have to put on a cheap suit and walk around in the big city, or cut the grass in the big city in the neighborhood where you aspire to live in, surround yourself with positivity and opportunities. Even if you have to buy three suits and walk around downtown with a smile on your face, buy them; you just never know what you're attracting. That just might be the day somebody walks up on you to ask what your occupation is. When you get to the end of the rope and you want to quit, that's a sign that you need to work on some things internally and figure out the why. Why is my confidence low? Why am I ready to give up? Why won't I give it one more try? Is it the voices in your head telling you to give up? Is it because your money is getting low, you don't have this, you don't have that, you've been through too much, you believe nothing ever works out anyway, or you're tired of fighting? If you're tired of fighting, then it's time for you to get back into the gym and strengthen your mental muscles to handle more pressure.

4. **Hospitality to all**: Treat everybody like the biggest thing in the world. Respect and appreciation will take you a long way in life. A homeless man walked up explaining why he needed me to give him money. I told him to save the stories and tell me how he planned on using the money to help better his situation. The conversation carried on for a few minutes as I explained to him how important his presence was to our society. I needed him to know, man to man, that regardless of his present situation, never to give up and never give excuses before I handed him ten dollars. The man smiled and appreciated me actually taking the time out to converse with him. Making this human being smile meant more to me than having the ability to give him money because I knew I

planted a seed. Planting this seed changed the dynamics of how the rest of his day, and hopefully his whole life, would be enhanced. I use this same concept in business as well. If you have a mentor taking the time out to benefit your future, show them your appreciation through how you value their time. Sometimes, treating a person to lunch, sending a thank you card, or any initiative to make the person feel special are examples of hospitality. By doing so, you are positioning yourself to receive greater blessings. This characteristic will also help some people eliminate themselves out of your life. Some people will get negative about your positive outlook on life and will show their true colors. When people don't show you that they're happy for you, that's when your association with them becomes a problem. Hospitality will help you decipher the right energy to maintain and conquer spiritual demons seeking to keep you down.

5. **Believe in something greater than yourself**: The beauty of different generations is the different walks of prayer life before us. At times people look at God as a resource versus being the actual source of their desires. Finding a healthy spiritual balance adjusts the way you handle your relationship with God. Once this is done, you can truly experience peace of mind in line with the creator. Now, money can be created because you're back in a positive space. When you're in a negative space, you can't attract money and opportunities because you have closed the

door and are no longer open to possibilities. How can you attract something when you're in isolation? If you hide yourself, you can't attract opportunities. It won't happen until you open yourself up, come out of that depression, and get into a space to attract opportunities. Ultimately, positivity attracts positive outcomes and people with positive energy usually have a positive life. In this world we live in, family, happiness, peace, contentment, and completion are usually the components that make people positive.

6. **Learn that different is great and powerful**: Everybody has something that's unique about themselves. Unfortunately, external influences such as marketing in the entertainment industry have blinded us from what is really taking place; hard work. We see the visuals of one person's success and begin to think, "Maybe I need to be more like that person." Pulling you further from who you were meant to become, you mold yourself to imitate someone you don't even know, including yourself. Many of us lose ourselves in this society. However, the most successful people in the world are the ones who remain true to themselves. Remember, everyone has something special about them and we shouldn't train ourselves to treat people differently based on their status or occupation.

7. **It's okay to pat yourself on the shoulder**: People who are successful are usually people who feel complete.

Hence, the purpose of setting goals to accomplish. A lot of people are stressed out and giving up simply because they are falling victim to the "feeling sorry for themselves" syndrome. You think there's no hope because the sun no longer shines on the other side of the mountain. When this happens, write down some of the things you would have done differently during that time you were in that space. After ten years of showing up late to work, they finally fired you because the time built up. If you get another opportunity, show up five minutes early to get ahead of the game. Now, you've put yourself in a position to not encounter fear, anxiety, worry, or depression because you're more prepared. Based on those things, celebrate when you complete at least one thing on that list. This shows growth and helps you to not fall short again.

8. **All in or nothing**: Beware of people who have one foot on their dreams and the other on their nine-to-five. There's a difference between having a side hustle and taking that leap of faith. A side hustle is a person who puts a little bit of money towards the dream in hopes it will manifest. A person with full faith takes everything they have to make things successful. Most of your top stars were homeless, fending for food and fighting to connect the dots every day. People told them to give up. Now, they are million to dang near billionaires because it wasn't a side hustle; they were all in. Even when you want to quit, still give it

one more try. Stop starting things that you don't intend to finish. And this time, take what you learn and figure out why it didn't work the first few times. Once you start to look at the reason why things didn't go right in your life, you'll begin to see how you played a part in your failure. The "why" forces us to take full responsibility. When I look back on my life with my group members, I had to evaluate all of the reasons why it didn't work out: selfishness, stubbornness, jealousy and pride. Most of the time when things go wrong, it's from negative emotions. This causes bad thoughts, which then lead to bad decisions. Instead of sticking together, one group member impatiently wanted more popularity than the other members. Ultimately, the fight for individual fame caused us to lose everything. Having a team is important because you can't be an expert in everything. However, it can also cause one's downfall if it isn't set with the right people. The team must be built on a strong foundation of loyalty and common ground in order to fulfill the mission. I believe there isn't one person on this earth who succeeded without the help of anyone. It's the team that breeds winners. Once you come to terms with this, the discovery of success is rewarding because it was accomplished with the people who understood the vision and were willing to share the task to reach it.

9. **Stay Gassed Up:** Life is like a car ride. The road is your path, the street signs are the messages of your direction,

and the lights are the pace of the journey. When traveling, make sure you have plenty of fuel in your tank, so your car won't cut off in the midst of accelerating or coming to a rest stop. This means to keep your mind and soul filled with positivity to keep from giving up when that red light happens in your life. The car is your body and the fuel is the energy used to keep you going. To get to your destination, the stop signs represent the challenges you will approach in order to excel to the next level. Remember, the great part about coming to a red light is knowing the green light is soon to follow. However, while you're waiting for the light to turn green, you must make sure you have the RIGHT fuel in your engine, so the negativity doesn't seep in and convince you that the light will never change. There is no such thing as having a smooth ride when embarking upon your purpose. You must have a few speed bumps to learn and adjust your route accordingly.

10. **Identify Yourself**: "They", are made of: Less versus Many. This is the same in our society. At the bottom it's crowded, full of the same type of people who are just surviving. The pigeons are the ones who eat whatever, scavenge for leftovers, and make ends meet. They are comfortable and usually living to pass time. An eagle is the survivor. This bird is a carnivore with no remorse when it comes to its appetite. The eagle is focused and only flies amongst other eagles; representing standards.

Jay-Z killed them when he said, "How high is high enough? Until we see eye to eye with the higher ups." If you are an eagle flying with pigeons, then you need to look up and realign your altitude. Eagles see eye to eye, while pigeons' dwell together. You won't find billionaires dwelling outside of their caliber of people because they don't want small minds rubbing on to them. They are always striving for more to remain at the top. Identify yourself through your circle. Pay close attention to those around you and reflect on their progression within the year. Once you recognize how they've grown, evaluate if they are flying at the same altitude that you aspire to soar. If you can identify complacency in their flight, then expect to fly as high as them. Attract greatness and your identity will reflect one and the same.

CHAPTER SIX

Miss Your Moment

Think about the last time you encountered a near death experience. Yes, these occurrences can be when someone rear ended you, the time when you were walking down the street and something fell off the roof almost hitting you, or when you were in the hospital and the doctors had to resuscitate you. But, have you truly had a near death experience? If you understood what I meant, then you would answer yes. You see, we all encounter people who are walking dead every day. Anyone can fall victim to being in this category; family, friends, loved ones, or even people you walk past on a daily basis. They are the people who are buried six feet above ground. Signs you are amongst the walking dead are the way you feel around them and the words they speak into existence. You could be having an amazing day and immediately feel drained when they come around. They may lack compassion, be ungrateful or even heartless. Although blood may flow through their veins and every organ works to keep them alive, beware of the people who are dead within. They no longer aspire for greatness, challenge themselves to reach the next altitude in life, and ultimately no longer have a desire for anything.

Anyone who dwells in the presence of a person who is walking dead can attest to encountering a near death experience. It is dangerous because it can easily be transferred onto you if your mind and spirit isn't grounded; doing so can cost you everything. People of this caliber put themselves in bad predicaments and miss their moment due to selfishness, lack of staying focused, or being blind to the fact that "now" is the right time. You can be the best singer in your group and begin to think everything revolves around you. Failing to realize your talent was put in place to impact millions, you miss your time. When this happens, it's hard to get that opportunity again. Then someone usually blows up right in your face, accomplishing the same task. If you want to bloom into your true being, you have to learn to get out of your own way. Did you know your past knows your future? They've actually met before. Whereas, the present you is the stranger. Your past knows your future is full of blessings. The enemy will fight you because he knows what's to come. These are called temptations; strongholds that must be broken.

Words are essential to time. It is when history is made and where every second is recorded. This is where I want to encourage you to remain humble and maximize the time of your present opportunities. I know it will be hard, but you have to fight hard not to allow negative energy to enter into your space. We live in a world where people are caught up in competing with the next person.

Instead of spending that energy thinking you can send emails better than your colleague, transfer your energy to complete the mission. Figuring out how to maximize your relationships is the key to fulfilling common goals. In this process you discover those who are the Finishers verses the Fugazies. People who are finishers are successful. They are the ones who overcome the impossible by using their brilliance and creativity to produce the vision that changes the world. In contrast, Fugazies disrupt positive energy and the flow of supernatural possibilities, they are the ones who focus their energy in the wrong things like thinking they can keep a calendar better organized than you. They are the distraction from the vision. When they approach you in life, remember to operate in the spiritual realm. They are merely there to withhold you from reaping the fruits of your labor.

The power of time is a beautiful process, yet most people never see life for what it really is. Life occurs in seasons. A woman carries a baby for nine months because it needs time to develop. Based on the time of her pregnancy, the season and surroundings of her environment impacts the growth of the child. It's the same thing when it comes to adults. People birth thoughts and ideas, but not everybody can birth creativity. We live in a world where people don't value others' brains anymore, they only value status. However, don't forget everything starts from the mind. Success is about having the ability to feel what's around you, to fuel ideas with positive energy and bind to people you are equally yoked to. Somebody thought about the computer, they didn't always exist. I love the stories of Steve Jobs and Bill

Gates because they made people appreciate their gift of discernment. They were just simple, weird men using their mind to build a team ready to cultivate their vision and make it come to life. These two men dropped out of college and used their ability to look into the future to create the corporate structure of their individual technology companies Apple, Inc. and Microsoft. Then, they received funding for an office and employed college students to further produce ideas such as the different departments, job titles and office locations. Can you imagine where the world would be if they allowed people to keep them from fulfilling their purpose?

Unfortunately, you may have family and friends who will get into your head and tell you to not do something or tell you to wait another year. Don't let them kill your blessings. In the world today, people are operating backwards and think blessings start externally. When really, blessings don't make sense and aren't presented the way we expect them to be. You never know who has come into your space to bless you. Keep this in mind: There's no such thing as little people, only people waiting to be empowered at the right moment. Because everyone has a story, always acknowledge the struggles and stripes of another person before wanting to belittle them.

When you get your big moment, use that time to align your brain with mother earth. The creator will then maneuver things in your favor. When this is done, the right people will come into your life and be driven to help the vision come to life.

Time is essential because it keeps record of every outcome. Everything happens the way it's supposed to happen, yet people mess up their time because they over-analyze everything. They forget everything starts in your mind. People go looking for things in the wrong place thinking they know everything. Nobody became successful based on structure. They became successful off of their vision to create a good product and acknowledging the right time to run with the vision. Ask yourself, can you run with the vision and what type of influences do you have in your circle to see the vision through? Some people turn against the people that gave them the vision, then turn to a new person to figure out the plan and shit on the person who believed in them the most. Once you kill the time of your opportunity, you deprive a blessing, which then leads to destruction. This reminds me of God versus scientists and atheists. I just don't understand it. Nothing just exists without a creator coming up with the concept of the planets and the purpose of everything we live in today. God orchestrated this whole movement. If the moon was to be removed, we would all shoot up into the sky over 2500 miles an hour. How does the sun know to sit there in space? The exact location in space, not too far or close, that would harm human life. Somebody placed that here and said, "Don't move." Somebody put the moon there to keep the water from moving. Somebody said this is going to be the DNA of a human being. We are surrounded by things we cannot see. Because we were made in God's likeness to be creators, man has the ability to be like God and create new ideas, build buildings and enhance technology. We can create everything.

The catch is to see the creation through and to not get lost in the logo. Change the way you view the world around you. Apple and Microsoft are not corporate companies, they are a thought that came to life.

CHAPTER SEVEN

The Gift

When I was younger, I remember walking into school and we would all wait in the cafeteria before the bell would dismiss us to start our day. At the sounds of the ring, everyone would disperse and I would have to walk the opposite direction. I was considered to have a learning disability and was enrolled in remedial courses or what the students would call DEC: *dumb education classes.* As I reflect on my childhood, I now wonder how was I the uneducated person when I was able to achieve more than the average individual coming from Baltimore. I got a chance to see the world and travel to Tokyo, Japan, whereas the children who were smarter than me never even leave the city or have somebody invest a million dollars in them. And to think, how could I have accomplished all of this if I was considered to be slow? It's not that I was dumb, it was merely the subjects taught didn't resonate with my spirit. I am a creative person and creatives tend to think outside of the box. Attending a school that taught common core education, my mind rejected their teachings because mentally I was far past that. My mind operated in a creative space and could not comprehend the matters I was being forced to learn. The curriculum of the public-school system is not geared towards cultivating a child's creativity and can limit how far their imagination can carry them. Instead, we feed them what we want them to know and give them homework to keep them busy. Most of these students won't even complete the homework because it involves doing work they have no interest in. The only way we can truly help our children in seeing success is by understanding who they want to become. I've learned when a child's creativity is downsized, educators will view them as incompetent, when really, they're fighting to manifest their gift.

It baffles me how many millionaires exist without college degrees versus the number of college graduates who make less than that amount a year. The difference between these two classes of people are them knowing what they want out of life. Millionaires know to follow their DNA and utilize the special talent God has given them. This is what makes them powerful because they nurture and feed their gifts. Not everybody can be the best writer or reader. However, millionaires know how to be the best version of themselves and empower people who want to do the same and be strong in the areas where they are not. This is where everyone has the potential of becoming great in who they are: their true self.

By changing the dynamics of education, we can stop teaching people the "basics" and start working with people to discover their purpose. We all know by now that communication is a major problem in today's society. Any counselor will tell you the reason why most relationships fail is because there is a lack of communication. Why not take this same approach in learning our children and understanding their gift? Instead of telling our kids how to learn a specific way, let's start learning how we can develop their interests by using the basic curriculum to adhere to their talents. For example, if a child wants to be a singer, show them how to use math to calculate the right pitch in their voice or to determine the levels of which they should engineer to create the perfect melody. Teach our future musicians science through chemistry to help them understand the psychological benefits of the endorphins that are released in their body when they're expressing themselves through their creativity. Use reading and writing to help them understand how to comprehend music note symbols and the beauty in using their words to combine metaphors with thoughts to give a new meaning to their feelings. Teachers should build partnerships with their students to work along with them versus feeding them whatever we want them to know. Partnerships build great communities, which later build wealth. Once we begin to readjust our way of connecting with the youth, this is when school will have a greater impact in their life and give children something to look forward to into their adult life.

There will always come a time to pass the baton to the next generation. As an expert in your gift, it is your responsibility to mentor and share knowledge with the youth. This includes giving wisdom, expressing personal experiences, and reminding them of how strong they are when they forget their own strength. Today, I am known as the best Branding Architect in the nation and can be an asset to anyone's entertainment and press career. At the top of the new year, I invited my mentee to visit New York City: the place that symbolizes freedom and liberty. She was fresh in her field and was eager to have real-life experiences in the media world. It was a city she'd always wanted to visit, but knew she wanted it to be under the right circumstances: to cultivate her vision and build her business. As a teacher, I didn't try to tell her things I wanted her to know. Instead, I listened to her, had her present her goals to me, then brought her to New York to begin giving her the hands-on training she needed to close deals, meet the right people, and fulfill her purpose in public relations, branding and networking her net worth. You see, sometimes you have to remove yourself to transform into who you want to become. By taking her out of her comfort zone and hometown, I was able to expose her to a different life and present the gift of opportunity. Most people think gifts always have to be tangible and something delivered in a box. However, the greatest gifts are the ones that don't have to be contained, so we can appreciate its value and never physically lose it. We have to remember that the act of thinking about getting someone a gift is greater than giving the gift. The joy is in the thought of them giving you a gift that overrides the actual gift. As educators, it is our job to ensure we are properly equipping our students with the right tools in order for them to be successful. This requires patience and actively listening to their heart's desires.

The spiritual side of this is that evil will try to prevent you from accomplishing your goals. These are the people who are usually stuck in who they are and will probably never reach their fullest potential. Beware of these individuals; they are the ones who feast on poison and will try to feed you their theories to make you doubt your purpose. When a man gets married, the wedding symbolizes the commitment made publicly. However, he was already married in his mind when he proposed to his soon-to-be wife. We must do the same when mingling our desires with our outcomes. When God unleashes your gift, he has already given you the tools and the right people in your life to ensure you are great. Yet, the commitment must be made in your mind before people can see the gift with their eyes.

CHAPTER EIGHT

A New Way to See Your Problems

Some people can't accept the fact of not remaining who they once were. It took me a lot of years to understand and come to terms with that after losing major success as an artist. I couldn't stop chasing the old high, the life I wanted back so badly. My ego steered every decision after that in hopes to fill the void of missing Motown. For a long time, I would put myself in deals I knew I shouldn't have involved myself into, but deep down, I was hoping it would be the big break I needed to put me back in the spotlight. At some point, we have to keep it real with ourselves. I was binding myself to a substantial-amount of contracts with people due to my naivety and selfish motives. I was digging myself a deeper hole until finally, I found satisfaction in realizing "the big moment" is just a collection of the many small moments. It's not uncommon to get caught up in having tunnel vision. Understanding the extent of each portion of the tunnel enhances your view of the prize at the end of it. I was going after big moments instead of falling back and looking at all of the smaller opportunities right in front of me. Once I valued the small moments, I was able to appreciate the larger moments that rebuilt my career.

Get off trying to be the old you and become a better you. If not, you will find yourself suffering from depression and anxiety, panic and frustration. It's like trying to shoot from zero to one hundred instead of gradually taking the moments that are building you up to surpass the one hundred-margin. The elevator is moving so fast that once you hit the top floor, everything feels like its crashing all at once. Jobs get lost, somebody betrays you, then you start tumbling down hard. I've learned in life that it's cool to start small. Get in deals even when it doesn't seem exciting and build from it. It's like getting into a relationship and wanting the baddest chick versus getting with a chick who had bad chick potential. However, you're not willing to do the work. You want to jump right in and get the trophy girl. Then you get home and she gets undressed, takes off all of her make up and realize that she's not as perfect.

Failure is the introduction of the humble beginnings to unstoppable success. Many people have convinced themselves that failure is a bad thing, when really it is the turning point to greatness. Think about a time in your life when you were pursuing a goal you really wanted to accomplish. Now, count the number of times it took to fulfill your desired outcome. Sometimes, this may require adjustments of your strategy or trying different techniques to achieve excellence. While doing so, know that failing the first time isn't the end of the world. Hence, the more you fail, the smarter, stronger and wiser you become. By the last attempt, your experience in failing will grant you more satisfaction and appreciation of that final "win" you've been aspiring for.

Life without failures means you don't have any mistakes to learn from. Mistakes give you the ability to make wise decisions based on the circumstance. This is why it's so important for college students to get internships prior to applying for that dream job. Employers want to hire someone with a few battle wounds; a person who has experience in facing adversity while executing the proper plans. A person who has bumped their head a few times will examine why something didn't go right and will enhance their next action plan. It's just like the person who created the electric car: there's no telling how many times he failed at constructing the car without gas before he finally heard the engine crank to start. Although he was being told no, each attempt was making him a clever problem-solver, and that much closer to influencing the world.

The advancement of intellect will equip you to excel in anything you put energy towards. However, you must be able to recognize when you've mentally advanced to the next level. One thing I've noticed is how ungrateful a lot of people are. You have some people who will pray for things, receive the answers to their prayers and still be unhappy with life. These are the people who chase after unfulfilled emotions from their childhood and don't see the blessings right before them. They are more concerned with looking successful, rather than actually being successful. With these types of people, there's no such thing as having enough. Good can happen all around them and they will still complain, wanting more. This in turn can cause the person to involve themselves in multiple tasks for the attention, rather than obtaining one goal at a time for the satisfaction of the blessing within completion.

You don't ever want to be a jack of all trades and a master of nothing. Sometimes we tend to bounce all over the place with our passions. One minute you're focused on building a brand, the next you're wanting to settle for a mediocre job. The bottom line is you're trying not to give up, but every decision you make gets you another step closer to losing it all. What's worse is the frustration that comes along with it. The problem is obvious and you want to fix it, but the solution is so far-fetched that it tempts you to give up. Everything looks the same. Your finances, friends, surroundings, and aspirations never developed because you never invested into the possibilities of growing. The sad part about it is how acceptable giving up has become. When you're surrounded by people and environments where lost hope lives, the veil before you will make your citizenship amongst the have nots seem like the best community to be a part of.

This makes me think about my friend who is no longer with us, Trina, who passed away from cancer. Thank you for being put here as a messenger to remind people how blessed they truly are and to enjoy life while they have it. People believe she died too soon, when really, she was put here for a shorter period of time as a reminder we all needed. In life, we run around chasing more and more, trying to do better and aim higher for the stars. At some point, you have to sit back and be thankful. In today's time, if we would just show gratitude, we would have less stress. Because so many sacrifices have been made to get you this far, always remember you're an overcomer. Sometimes you have to switch the prescription of your glasses in order to get a better perception of life. Things will continue to look the same if we can't identify the source of the distraction. This is when you have to find a new way to "see" your problems and figure out the common denominator in each of the difficulties at hand. Once the common denominator is identified, map out how you intend to tackle it in order to give it one more try. We must first stop playing the victim and take ownership in the challenge. Throughout the process of your awakening, cultivate your understanding of how God is trying to manifest your purpose. This will sometimes require isolation.

CHAPTER NINE

The Power of Opportunity

My mother always said "All you need is one opportunity." What people confuse about opportunity is thinking they need several opportunities to lead up to their ultimate goal. When people are praying, asking God for a sign, there's always been that perception the sky will open up with strikes of lightning and his voice will announce "Here's your opportunity." When really, opportunities are delivered in the form of human life and God places the right person in your life to give you a chance to fulfill your destiny. In order to reach that certain level of success, you have to be invited. You can't just walk into a VIP event; somebody had to put you on the guestlist. You can't just walk into the VP office of your dreams and set up the desk because you want to; somebody had to offer the position to you. Because successful people dwell amongst each other, remember it only takes one invitation to the table of opportunity to meet that one person who will open the door for you, change the dynamics of your network, and impact your life.

Meeting the right person allows you to enter into a different realm that you wouldn't typically be involved in. Just as most upper-class families' children are born into riches, most people have to find their way to that "right" person. This requires stepping outside of your comfort zone to make the necessary steps towards the life you crave. Networking is key. Once you enter into that room to network, you will then be in a space of possibilities. With that, growth follows.

As you grow into your purpose, you will begin to desire to understand the consciousness you are accessing. The doors of accomplishment will open up to you as you feen for more knowledge and persevere through challenges. This is where the phrase "focus and follow" is key. Because trials are meant to evolve your existence and elevate your understanding, it is important to focus on the ultimate goals set before you. Remember that trials are merely roadblocks to the success in life you want to create. Once you are grounded in your calling, following your purpose will be worth the hardships. In addition, appreciating the timing of your chance is equally important. When a sixteen-year-old is presented an opportunity, they go after it because there's no fear of losing anything. They're living with their parents, being provided for, and in the sweet spot of their life of figuring everything out. At this age, everything appears differently because the mindset isn't fully developed and hasn't come to know the power of responsibility. You're free of children or having to support yourself. In contrast, when you're twenty-five, the mindset operates in an overanalyzing circumference and responsibilities open the door to skepticism. Although you have the ability, wisdom and/or experience to reach your full potential, now more distractions have been placed before you to challenge your endurance. This is where we give too much power to bills, materialistic desires and the accomplishments of others keeping us from solely focusing on what's superior to prevail in your mission. Be encouraged and always be logical in how you view the surface of your situation, so that you are not distracted by unrealistic expectations.

Let's take it back to the basics. In order to fulfill your destiny, you have to realize that an empire is never built overnight. To develop the body from the womb, it takes nine to ten months. To proceed from an adolescent to an adult, it takes fourteen years of education to earn a high school diploma. To be considered an expert in your field of major, it takes four years to obtain a bachelor's degree. The common denominator in all of this is the process of discipline, focus, and motivation to see the end results. School teaches the art of completion. Through the many tasks you are given, satisfaction comes when you are able to advance to the next level. This why it is important to finish what you start and to use this same concept as adults to become successful. Unfortunately, we become so happy to be done with school that we forget to use those tools when enhancing our skills and learning capabilities in life. However, the people who continue to complete each level of progress are the ones who advance in life. Just like in school, you have to study material given to you in order to pass a test.

Because this is a formula that has been taught our whole life, we must never forget to use these strategies when working towards success. When learning, you had consistent homework and assignments due on a weekly basis to constantly enhance your abilities in understanding the subject taught. Even when it was hard to comprehend and you felt like giving up, you knew the only way you could pass to the next grade is by proving you deserved to excel to the level. Take this same approach and patience when investing in your dreams. Break your life into phases, so that you are not trying to take on so much at once. By doing this, you will appreciate each milestone you accomplish along the way. Many people get discouraged because they are trying to master their plan in a short amount of time. When realistically, you must evaluate what is worth devoting your time to, visualize the plan of execution, then take the time to cultivate your masterpiece.

We live in an addiction driven society where people are chasing something to make them feel high. The majority of people think becoming successful is fun when really it takes self-control. I can talk all day about wanting to write a book, but never put pressure on myself to work on it. Eventually, the momentum dies and I could easily move on to something else as if this wasn't something I wanted to achieve. Most of the time, people will talk about starting something they do not attempt to finish. However, I was determined to finish this book because I knew it was going to impact the lives of many if I could just share my testimony with you. Once you thrive in these phases of your life, you will then become rich in accomplishments. This will lead to riches in happiness, then financial gain will follow.

CHAPTER TEN

Candice

Every person has a Candice in their life. Whether we pay attention and can identify who that person is, he or she is the reminder of strength, hope, perseverance, triumphs, struggle, determination and faith. Indirectly or directly, we've all come across that one person who has had a very challenging life more excruciating than our own personal problems. If we pay attention, we'll be able to see how God is always present through their existence. They are proof that anything is possible. This is who Candice is to me.

God places certain people in our lives for a particular reason and a lot of times, we just live our life on a day-to-day basis. Blind to the daily blessings we have been anointed with, our tunnel vision of focusing on self is keeping us from appreciating the people in our surroundings. These people have been put in place to teach us something more than what we could ever learn in school. This lesson is to acknowledge the fact of not being the only person with problems in the world. People like Candice make you stop and look around to see what others are going through. Bad things happening to other people can sometimes be a blessing to others. It challenges us to live through a different lens and appreciate the simple things in life like family, health, and opportunities.

My sister Candice is one of the strongest people I've met in life. Born with Neurofibromatosis (NF1), I can remember watching her as a young child having the might of a lion with the presence of an angel. As a baby, I would sometimes go check on her in the crib and find her shaking. Nobody knew what it was at the time. You have to remember this was back in the '90s, where resources were limited and access to the internet hardly existed. We were unaware of what it meant to have a seizure, but all my mom knew was she needed to seek extra help for Candice who was very young at this time. I remember seeing the disappointment on my mom's and stepdad's faces after repeatedly being given misinformation, and we were forced to cope with our bewilderment at her condition. My sister had a few seizures and developed spots all over her body. Running up the medical bill, my mom and stepdad took her to the doctor several times, just for the "experts" to give a million wrong reasons as to what was causing these problems. Thank God my stepfather had great health insurance and we were a praying family. Each trip back home from the doctor was futile, so we were forced to take things into our own hands. We began to sterilize everything, thinking maybe she had an incurable infection. Years later, the doctor informed us that the optical nerve in her eye had a tumor on it. While we had been searching for the right diagnosis, her eye was getting weaker and weaker. By this time, Candice has lost the sight in her eye.

As I reflect on the multiple doctor's visits and the fear of the unknown, these were the most confusing moments for all of us. Discovering her diagnosis of NF1 was the hardest day of acceptance, but also a provided feeling of relief for our family because we were finally given the right answer after being told the wrong diagnosis for so long. From that day on, everything revolved around my sister's health. As she grew older, she began to notice her own imperfections. I remember when the doctors recommended that Candice wear braces for her spine, so it wouldn't bend as she developed into her teenage years. The spots on her body began to progress aggressively, so she had to accept the discoloration of her skin. Her seizure medication was strong and prevented her from going outside into the sun. All of these symptoms were stressful, as was the fact that she constantly needed MRIs and body examinations. However, we remained faithful, knowing God would help us during these challenging moments.

Candice is so precious to us. Collectively, our family was cautious of every change to her life. As she grew older, she not only had to deal with this condition every day, but now she had to face other children at school who appeared to be "normal." This then led to some self-esteem issues because she was conscious about her appearance. No matter how badly we wanted to protect her from the world, we knew we couldn't shelter her and prevent her from getting an education. Unfortunately, she had to deal with the awkward stares and questioning with one eye appearing different from the other eye. Some days were tougher than others. At one point, she would cry so hard to me, begging me not to make her go. As her big brother, I wanted to save her. I knew she was looking to me to be her blanket. I felt like the worst person because I couldn't go to school with her each and every day.

Taking her to school, it was battle to get her out of the car as we talked for the longest few minutes, building her courage and strength. There were times when after she would finally get out of the car, I would sit in the parking lot and cry: thanking God for making her so strong just for getting out of the car, but wishing I could've done more for her. The days when she would call me for comfort were essential because I knew she wanted to quit, but she knew it wasn't an option.

Every person comes to a point where they question God and simply want to give up on themselves. This was my Candice many times during her college experience. Eventually, she felt like there was no reason to keep trying. Sometimes, she had terrible headaches and all we could give her was Tylenol. Everything and everyone in our surroundings affected Candice's wellbeing.

You see, the average person is concerned with how good they look in their designer clothes, while there are people struggling to feel good in the skin they are in. I watched a little girl from birth having the worries and pressure of her own existence in this very world we share. While the average person expects to wake up every day on the right side of the bed, imagine being Candice, not knowing what the new challenges of the day or the next hour may bring. I say this because I want you to appreciate the fact that some people were placed here on this earth to focus more on the awareness of their health rather than the distractions of the world placed before us classified as "problems". A person who's never had these challenges wouldn't understand the trials of a person who lives a health-driven lifestyle. Remember, there is always someone who has a few more obstacles that you do, so never take your life for granted.

I am more than proud of my sister because she was able to do something that most people struggle to do; keep going. Being so close to giving up, we can welcome her to the next chapter of her life because we understood her journey and the courage it took to arrive there. Her graduation wasn't the typical graduation of watching her cross the stage for her high school diploma, it was a celebration of triumph and her will to overcome life's obstacles. On the day she went to college, tears of joy flowed from my face because I *knew* she truly deserved to be right where she was. Regardless of what she endured, she refused to stop. We live in a world where some people have never been through tribulations and quit when one thing goes wrong. My sister is the definition of "give it one more try." When she was exhausted and consumed with negativity, she continued to give it one more try.

In her adult years, Candice began to have panic attacks because she carried loads of anxiety from school and the negative relationship of our parents. This constant battle led to being admitted to a psychiatric hospital for a whole week because the panic attacks had consumed her mind. Although her physical wellbeing was questioned, we knew this was another hurdle Candice would overcome. I feel people who are strong and have purpose in fulfilling God's plan will be given great tasks in life. Regardless of the attacks formed, Candice was fighting with all of her might…and was winning. We had people across the nation praying for my sister and with every visit to the mental institution, I saw Candice coming back to us. Despite the situation, her life brought the family closer because all we had was each other, faith and hope. We all began to go to church together, pray together and, sooner rather than later, we healed together.

All of a sudden, Candice woke up and it all stopped. Candice snapped out of everything and was back to herself like nothing ever happened. She was now home and her spirit shined brightly. She would watch the Trinity Broadcasting Network all the time, and all I could hear was "be patient during the process of prayer." God validated his power in our lives by using my sister as a testimony. She had been restored completely and ever since then, she's been giving life one more try.

Seeing my sister go through these hurdles brought me closer to God and encouraged me to face my own battles. I was placed in a position where my faith and perspective on life was strengthened. Everything that I've experienced and have been a witness to has shown me that with man this is impossible, but with God all things are possible. In life, we can pick and choose our battles, but we can never choose the war. No matter what you go through, always remember the value in giving yourself one more try at whatever you are seeking to accomplish. This is because, you are not only doing yourself a favor, but you are being a living testimony to a person who is witnessing you persist in the face of your hardships. There are so many people who are just one second away from risking it all, yet you could give them hope just from hearing your story. You are blessing someone else through your dedication.

Today, I want to inspire you to find the Candice in your life who has been through more than you, yet overcame the worst. The moment you feel like giving up, identify that person, look at their situation versus yours, then ask yourself, "Is it worth losing it all?" For this person to be so close in your circle, this means you have the same abilities to accomplish just what they did. It's the same thing when you see a person getting off the disability bus in a wheelchair to go inside of the grocery store, or the person swimming in the pool with you with no legs, or even the person who has cancer sitting next to you in the doctor's office. Regardless of the facts, they chose to keep living. If you were to quit now, would you be a part of the discouragement or the hope of people's lives? When things get rough, think outside of yourself and search for that Candice in your life and in your surroundings as an example of what God can do for you.

CHAPTER ELEVEN

Design

After running in circles, I finally took a moment to breathe and ingest the truth placed within me from birth. As I reflect on my childhood, I think about the different personalities which pinpointed exactly who I was going to be. I was very emotional, compassionate towards others, appreciative of every situation, and inquisitive about life and the world we live in. At the age of thirteen, I was intrigued by the Bible and the interpretations of our existence. At fifteen, I began studying books that taught the depths of life and experiences. By the time I was seventeen, my mind exuded thought-provoking conversations that made adults embrace my knowledge and old soul. I knew then my passion was to empower people by building self-awareness and to assist those seeking solutions.

God gives each one of us special gifts and talents. Many times, we don't tap into our gifts because we allow our desires to distract us. For example, I spent many years wanting to become the next Michael Jackson. I knew that if I was the best singer and dancer, I would be famous and live the "American Dream." However, everyone saw me as a visionary and helpmate in my day-to-day life. I began to lose myself when I tried to utilize my gifts in the wrong way to obtain these desires. The wrong intentions set the tone for making wrong decisions and allowing the wrong energy into my space. This only suffocated my gifts because they were fighting to be highlighted in an environment it didn't belong in. I began to recognize the patterns in my life and acknowledge where the stress was stemming from. Then it all connected; I was stressing because I was doing things pushing me against my purpose, which caused me to grow emptier the more I chased the "high." The moment I began to operate in my gift for the right reason, I saw the rewards in building people and their brands. I wasn't only motivating them on how to make adjustments in their life, but I was coaching myself on how to heal by seeing the good in every bad situation. I was finding myself, and my purpose, by tuning into my gift.

One day, Candice asked me "What does it mean when God says he won't put more on you than you can bare?" The innocence in her voice in what seemed like the simplest question made me think about the airplane. Meteorologists predict the weather all the time and based on the forecast, airports determine if it's safe for their passengers to travel in the air. From a distance, the sky looks clear and the clouds are positioned perfectly to provide the best visual and flight experience. When it's time to take off, unexpected turbulence takes place and it's too late to turn back because you're already in motion. You make it through the hard part and just as the meteorologist said, there was clear skies and the pleasant experience as promised. Just as the airplane was designed to withstand the turbulence, it's the same thing in life. God designed you to succeed and to handle everything that comes along with it. You were already equipped mentally, emotionally and physically to endure the journey and overcome the worst.

Because this is true, the enemy will try to discourage and distract you from what you were placed on earth to do. Instead of facing these trials, many people reach for drugs, sex, or alcohol to find an escape. Today is the day you stop reaching outside of your gifts for temporary fixes. Remember, where there is a will, there's a way, so never give up on finding the answers within yourself.

25 Quotes To Live By

Don't block your success

School teaches the art of completion

Make the decision to live

Speak life into your life

Beware of your circle of influence

Only you can unlock your destiny to freedom

The truth is the padlock on the
door and you are the key

Find the willpower to open the
door to prosperity

Don't give into depression and anxiety

Fight for your existence

Be patient during the process of prayer

Cultivate your understanding in how
God is trying to manifest your purpose

Believe in something greater
than yourself

Different is great and powerful

Cope with fear

The team must be built on a strong foundation
in order to breed winners

You are giving the next person hope
just from hearing your story

You never know what lies ahead
in not giving up

To settle is to undervalue yourself

Your bank account is a reflection
of your state of mind

You don't need more money,
you need a better strategy

With division, comes weakness

The most dangerous person to face is yourself

Limitations groom creativity

Proper planning prevents poor preparation

GIVE IT ONE MORE TRY

JOURNAL

Remember Why You Started

List 5 things that are important to you

1) _____

2) _____

3) _____

4) _____

5) _____

It All Starts With Gratitude

List 10 Things You are Grateful For

1) _____

2) _____

3) _____

4) _____

5) _____

6) _____

7) _____

8) _____

9) _____

10) _____

The Joy of the Lord is Your Strength

List 5 Things That Bring You Joy

1) _____

2) _____

3) _____

4) _____

5) _____

Life Gets Tough Sometimes

What Obstacles are You Currently Facing?

_____

_____

_____

_____

_____

_____

_____

_____

_____

_____

Trials Will Come, Anticipate Them and Prepare

List 5 Things You Can Do to Overcome

1) _____

2) _____

3) _____

4) _____

5) _____

Personal Daily Reflections

Personal Daily Reflections

Personal Daily Reflections

Personal Daily Reflections

_____

_____

_____

_____

_____

_____

_____

_____

_____

_____

_____

_____

_____

Personal Daily Reflections

_____

_____

_____

_____

_____

_____

_____

_____

_____

_____

_____

_____

Personal Daily Reflections

Personal Daily Reflections

Personal Daily Reflections

_____

_____

_____

_____

_____

_____

_____

_____

_____

_____

_____

_____

_____

Personal Daily Reflections

_____

_____

_____

_____

_____

_____

_____

_____

_____

_____

_____

Personal Daily Reflections

Personal Daily Reflections

Personal Daily Reflections

Personal Daily Reflections

_____

_____

_____

_____

_____

_____

_____

_____

_____

_____

_____

Personal Daily Reflections

_____

_____

_____

_____

_____

_____

_____

_____

_____

_____

_____

Personal Daily Reflections

_____

_____

_____

_____

_____

_____

_____

_____

_____

_____

_____

Personal Daily Reflections

_____

_____

_____

_____

_____

_____

_____

_____

_____

_____

_____

_____

_____

Personal Daily Reflections

_____

_____

_____

_____

_____

_____

_____

_____

_____

_____

_____

Personal Daily Reflections

Personal Daily Reflections

Personal Daily Reflections

Personal Daily Reflections

_____

_____

_____

_____

_____

_____

_____

_____

_____

_____

_____

_____

Personal Daily Reflections

Personal Daily Reflections

_____

_____

_____

_____

_____

_____

_____

_____

_____

_____

_____

_____

Personal Daily Reflections

Personal Daily Reflections

_____

_____

_____

_____

_____

_____

_____

_____

_____

_____

_____

_____

Personal Daily Reflections

_____

_____

_____

_____

_____

_____

_____

_____

_____

_____

_____

_____

_____

Personal Daily Reflections

Personal Daily Reflections

Personal Daily Reflections

_____

_____

_____

_____

_____

_____

_____

_____

_____

_____

_____

_____

Personal Daily Reflections

_____

_____

_____

_____

_____

_____

_____

_____

_____

_____

_____

_____

_____

Personal Daily Reflections

_____

_____

_____

_____

_____

_____

_____

_____

_____

_____

_____

_____

Personal Daily Reflections

Personal Daily Reflections

_____

_____

_____

_____

_____

_____

_____

_____

_____

_____

_____

_____

Personal Daily Reflections

Personal Daily Reflections

Personal Daily Reflections

Personal Daily Reflections

Personal Daily Reflections

Personal Daily Reflections

_____

_____

_____

_____

_____

_____

_____

_____

_____

_____

_____

Personal Daily Reflections

Personal Daily Reflections

Personal Daily Reflections

Personal Daily Reflections

Personal Daily Reflections

_____

_____

_____

_____

_____

_____

_____

_____

_____

_____

_____

_____

_____

Personal Daily Reflections

Personal Daily Reflections

Personal Daily Reflections

Personal Daily Reflections

Personal Daily Reflections

Personal Daily Reflections

_____

_____

_____

_____

_____

_____

_____

_____

_____

_____

_____

_____

Personal Daily Reflections

Personal Daily Reflections

_____

_____

_____

_____

_____

_____

_____

_____

_____

_____

_____

_____

_____

_____

Personal Daily Reflections

Personal Daily Reflections

Personal Daily Reflections

CPSIA information can be obtained
at www.ICGtesting.com
Printed in the USA
BVHW010628151120
593359BV00003B/17

9 781734 179729